A Child

Is a Terrible

Thing to Waste

BY QUEEN ZAKIA SHABAZZ

United Parents Against Lead & Other Environmental Hazards

For Zaki

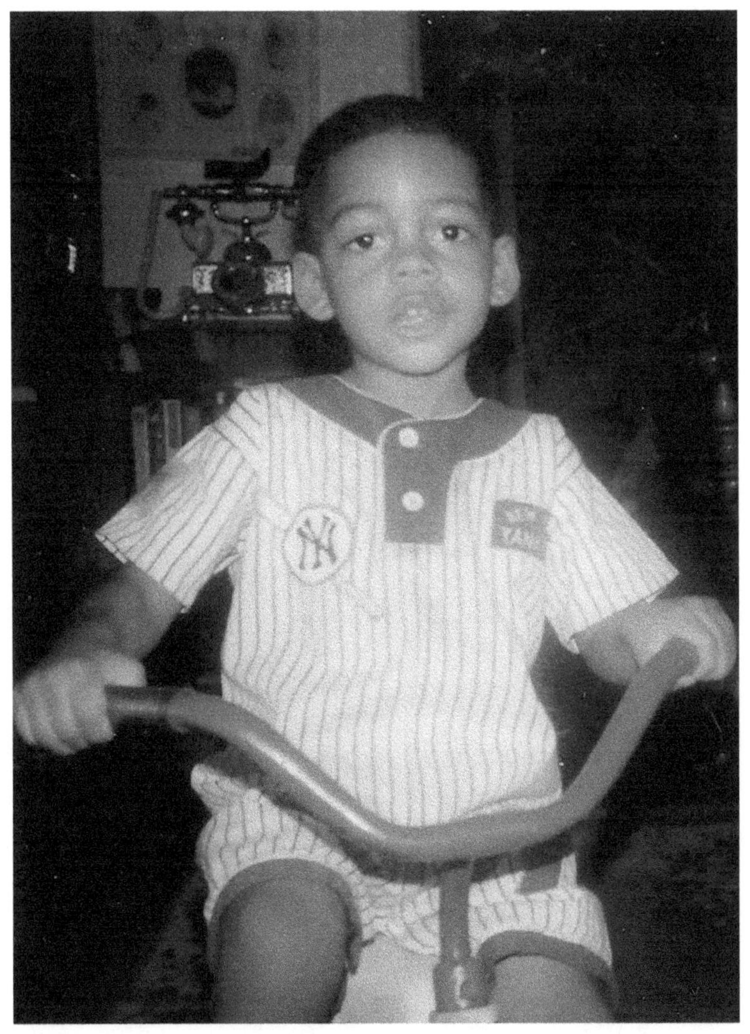

Dedications To

My loving mother Margaret who
is my source of inspiration,

Maurci Jackson, my comrade in the struggle
who had the courage to stand alone,

Maura Jackson - Mother of Maurci Jackson,
a trusted friend and confidant,

Seshem't Saa, Clara Tolbert, Shonta Reid,

Sister Friends who remind me that
my odds depend on me,

Cynthia Mendy, who will always have
my mutual support and respect,

The many, many lead poisoning
prevention advocates around the world
who fight this fight every day,

All the parents of lead poisoned children
who have decided to scream out
against environmental injustice,

All UPAL chapters – United We Stand!

Marian Wright Edleman for taking
a STAND FOR CHILDREN,

Lastly and Mostly to Lead Poisoned Children
Everywhere, know that when you are told
to "be seen and not heard," there are many
voices speaking out on your behalf.

I have much love for all of you and pray that you
receive continuous blessings of strength and clear
vision. You have enriched my life immeasurably.

Thanks for Being

Special Mention and Thanks To

Steve Larue Shabazz, my everything and more. Special, special, special, special thanks to **Rafiqa, Aqua, Radiah and Messiah Shabazz.** My children who so graciously share their mother with the rest of the world, never once complaining and always understanding that **WE** are doing this for **Zaki**. Thanks for your hugs, kisses, encouraging words and unquestionable love.

A Posthumus Thanks to **Sylvina Poole**, my trusted editor/publisher, sister friend. I appreciate you traveling on this journey with me.

Look at how we have grown!

Contents

Foreword

By Sylvina Poole

People who believe, 'the darkest hour is just before dawn,' must have read my mind. This old proverb means that just before the sun rises, the sky is at its blackest, suggesting when times are at their worst for us, they will soon get better.

The sun shone unseasonably brighter the day I met Queen Zakia Shabazz for the first time. I did not know it then, but it would be a sure sign of things to come. What I experienced in the coming days, and decades later learned, is she would bring the light with her even in some of the darkest times of my life. Her premier book, ***A Child Is a Terrible Thing to Waste*** is a testimony to that end in how she is able to turn life-altering despair into a tapestry of triumph and purpose.

Queen single-handedly creates a platform for herself to stand on and a voice to those experiencing issues with lead-poisoning and other environmental hazards. In her premier book, she chronicles her life experience nurturing a lead-poisoned child and how it impacted her family. She proved to the world that she would not stand idly by as a victim but rather a force to be reckoned with **all day, snap, snap!**

Far greater than a captivating story of overcoming obstacles, ***A Child Is a Terrible Thing to Waste*** gives life lessons and anecdotal remedies that help the reader to overcome pain and darkness in their own lives. Even more so, the reader obtains a clear understanding of ways to pick up the pieces, gaining strength to go on in their own lives.

Decades later, after our initial introduction, Queen Zakia Shabazz has become a sister, mentor, an unshakable spiritual force, and visionary guide, lighting the way to my path and others. ***A Child Is a Terrible Thing to Waste*** is a must read for anyone looking to learn how to overcome hurdles and challenges as they navigate life's journey.

For anyone who has been through any life struggle, this book is for you and serves as a model for inspirational lessons providing a platform for tools necessary through any struggle. Queen Shabazz is the official "Sojourner Truth" of lead awareness and environmental dangers.

A Child Is a Terrible Thing to Waste is a page-turner for anyone looking for inspiration to overcome life's challenges and persevere successfully.

Author and advocate Queen Shabazz has written an immensely powerful book about her son's struggle to survive a life-threatening battle with lead poisoning that is one of a few of its kind ever penned until now.

This is one of the first books ever written which gives a first-hand look at this deeply traumatic experience.

A must-read for all parents, children advocates, health organizations, and lead poisoning prevention groups.

Shabazz had lifted the veil from the preventable health issue of childhood lead poisoning. She currently lives her day continuing to fight the cause for other families, giving them voice, support, and inspiration. She travels across the country giving speeches and workshops, telling audiences about her personal experience, and serving as a valuable resource to victims.

Queen Shabazz allows the reader an in-depth peek into her world of undergoing one of the most traumatic experiences in her life of saving a child. ***A Child Is a Terrible Thing to Waste*** is a soul-searching book that resonates with many people on the power of love and perseverance. One can learn a great deal from the truthful lessons in ***A Child Is a Terrible Thing to Waste*** and apply them the next time confronted with a challenge in their own personal journey.

I have often shared with her how much knowledge and value I have personally gained from her in taking the high road on many matters. She does not just talk the talk. She walks the walk every step of the way. To Queen, I say, I have learned respect, admiration, countless lessons, and most of all the true meaning of STRENGTH. Thanks for being authentic and sharing this with others. Congratulations on another job well done. Keep shining your light, my sister.

Introduction

During the early 1970s I went along with family members to visit my younger cousin, Tony, in a hospital in Brooklyn, New York.

Tony was very young and very bad off. He had eaten paint chips. Paint chips laced with lead. He was dreadfully weak and in the intensive care unit. I remembered his eyes had crossed. I was about eleven years old.

We all prayed for him and eventually he recovered (got well enough to be released from the hospital not recovered in the sense of being free from the ravages of lead) but the lead had done its damage. The irreversible damage to his brain has left him unable to be a "contributing member of society." As a little girl I knew that something terrible had happened to him. At eleven years old, I had no way of knowing that years later lead would again visit our family.

Only this time in 1996 it hit much closer to home. This book is written with hopes and prayers that your children and loved ones can be spared the devastating harm caused by lead poisoning. We share our experience as a family who battled lead poisoning and WON.

BOOK I

Pb

Pb is the symbol for lead - Lead is a heavy metal. Lead is a deadly element that should never enter the body for lead offers absolutely no beneficial value to the human body.

Lead poisoning is the number one environmental threat to young children.

Chapter 1

Exposure to Lead
During Pregnancy

Lead is all around us, thus I feel it appropriate to start at the beginning and discuss lead poisoning during pregnancy. A large percentage of childhood lead poisoning is passed on to unborn babies through the placenta. During pregnancy all heavy metals should be avoided.

These include cadmium, manganese, nickel, and, of course, lead. Even a little lead is too much for the immature, undeveloped brain. Heavy exposure to lead can put a woman at increased risk of developing pregnancy-induced hypertension, and at higher risk to miscarry.

Some women who need calcium supplements may use bone meal or oyster shell tablets. These are high in lead, cadmium, mercury and other toxic metals. Among the most potent poisons are mercury and dioxins. While my focus is on lead, you, the reader, are urged to learn as much as you can about these other harmful toxins as well. Every year over one billion pounds of toxic chemicals are released into the environment in the United States.

A pregnant woman with lead in her body can pass it to her baby. Lead is known to cause lasting harm to the brain and other organs. This is especially true to an undeveloped fetus. Studies show that lead can effect an unborn baby's developing brain and nervous system before birth. That child most likely will have learning and behavioral problems and may have a lower intelligence quotient (IQ) in comparison with other children of the same age. These problems can last a lifetime. Pregnant women exposed to lead are at high risk of giving birth prematurely. Premature birth in turn increases the risk for illnesses and death. Low birth weight babies are sometimes the result of exposure to lead. Babies that are too small at birth also face a higher risk of illness and death. Many unborn babies can't survive the very High levels of lead exposure and are stillborn (born dead).

The placenta or umbilical cord supplies oxygen and nutrients to the unborn baby from the mother. We know that everything a pregnant woman ingests is shared with the unborn baby. Thus the poisoning of the child is like a chain reaction. A pregnant woman breathes in or swallows lead. The lead enters her blood stream. The lead passes through the placenta and gets into the baby's brain, bones and other vital organs. Lead is like a leech. Remember the leeches used in olden days for medicinal purposes? Leeches are blood sucking worms. Lead is like a leech because lead will store itself in a young woman's bones and remain there for years. When that woman becomes pregnant and needs minerals that are stored in the bones, lead is released along with the minerals back into the woman's bloodstream and is passed through the placenta to the baby. An estimated 90% of the lead stored in the mother's body is free to cross the placenta to the fetus. It is also important to be aware that lead can pass through breast milk. It can build up to high levels in breastfed infants. The vicious cycle continues.

There are often no symptoms of low level exposure in adults. If there are symptoms they most often are not attributed to lead and are mistaken for other illnesses. These may include headaches, mood changes, fatigue, abdominal pain and anemia. Some of us women experience these on a daily or monthly basis. I myself was anemic during all six of my pregnancies. Not once was I tested for lead. While lead poisoning was not passed on to my son through pregnancy many of our children are poisoned in this way. I strongly urge women of child bearing age to have yourselves tested for lead.

Test before and during pregnancy. Maurci Jackson who is the Founder of Parents Against Lead has a daughter who was exposed before birth. Her other daughter was exposed during renovation of their Chicago residence. Both had elevated blood lead levels, both experienced diminished capacities. Both instances could have been prevented.

History of Lead

Lead has been around forever. Its use goes back several decades. "White lead", aggressively promoted as the best protective coating that provided long, economical surface protection, was used not only on interior and exterior walls of homes but was also used on baby cribs, toys, and furniture. It is estimated that three million tons of lead still coats the walls and woodwork of American homes.

The first U.S. case of child lead poisoning was reported in 1914. This resulted from lead carbonate paint better known as white lead. In 1922, it was discovered that tetraethyl lead improved the performance and efficiency of automobiles. The lead industry touted lead as the "Gift of God." Now, in addition to leaded homes, cribs and toys children had to contend with leaded automobile exhaust. The lead industry launched a medical and political campaign to ensure that the use of lead not be restricted. This campaign was so effective and so heavily funded that it still exists today. Through the 1920s, the National Bureau of Standards (NBS) consistently recommended white lead for use in schools. Thanks to the lead industry's unscrupulous business methods, the federal government estimates about 15% of all U.S. preschoolers now have unacceptable levels of lead in their blood, levels that cause subtle but significant impairment of learning skills.

Back then (1922) a Yale University physiologist issued warnings that the leaded automobile exhaust fumes emitted a poisonous dust. The lead industry won over the warnings and during the next half-century about 7 million tons of lead entered the air from automobile exhaust. We breathe this air. All the while the lead industry provided funds to medical experts who asserted that lead exposure was harmless and normal. Meaningful regulation continued to be thwarted as the industry gained control over the conduct of medical research and set the tone of public health priorities including the dissemination of information and warnings to the public. Manufacturers continuously disputed claims of lead poisoning. Moreover, in 1930 when the introduction of non-toxic paints provided unwanted competition, the lead industry worked diligently to assure that lead paint would be required in public housing projects and other public buildings. This is no surprise. I personally know of several children who have been poisoned while living in public housing, most owned and operated by the U.S.

Department of Housing and Urban Development (HUD).

In April 1990, HUD issued the first federal guidelines for abatement of lead-based paint in public housing.

Although the lead industry also provided bullets and pipe, paint was still its most viable product. The industry claimed that lead surpassed all other substances as paint and because of its malleability it was prized as a conduit for water (thus it's even present day use in pipes). Mines, smelters and refineries grew in vast numbers, as lead became a powerful force in the nation's economy. The largest lead-producing district in the United States was in southeastern Missouri. Oftentimes when we hear about industry or large plants moving into our area we are always guided by the media to think that it is a good thing in terms of employment and gain for the community. The health issues are almost never discussed until the numbers of miscarriages, damaged children and ailing workers start to mount. Then it is usually too late. The damage has been done and billions of dollars have been made. On the backs of the poor and voiceless. For two thousand years the dangers of lead have been known to cause disease and death yet it is used where it is most dangerous. Environmental racism is indeed another form of industrialized discrimination.

As early as 1920 European nations ratified the ban on the use of white lead. In the United States the National Paint, Oil and Varnish Association successfully opposed the ban and the use of lead continued to the detriment of our children. In America, cash is usually chosen over conscience.

Lead Blockers

Calcium

It is important for both the pregnant woman and the unborn child that the mother partakes of calcium. Calcium is a mineral that is beneficial to women before, during and after pregnancy. Calcium acts as a lead blocker. In cases where lead had entered the teeth and bones there was a lack of sufficient calcium. My son Zaki's teeth suffered the most damage from his lead exposure and are discussed in further detail in Chapter Four.

Lack of calcium during pregnancy attributes to muscle cramps, backache, high blood pressure, intense labor and afterbirth pains, osteoporosis, and tooth problems. Women need 1000 to 2000 mg of calcium daily whether pregnant or not. Good food sources of calcium are fish and dairy products. Highly recommended are salmon, seaweed, tahini, and dark, green leafy vegetables. Many fruits are also rich in calcium: dried dates, figs, raisins, prunes and papayas are good sources.

Recipes

Children will enjoy these while getting a boost of calcium and iron:

Fruit Kabob - 10 minutes

Ingredients:

1 ½ cups banana, sliced
1 ½ cups watermelon, cubed
1 cup clementine sections

Thread the fruit sections onto skewers alternating and arranging them in a pattern of your choice.

Serve right away or place in the refrigerator until ready to serve.

Apple and Celery Salad - 15 minutes

1 tablespoon orange juice
2 tablespoons light mayonnaise
2 cups apples, diced
1 cup celery, diced
½ cup raisins

In a large bowl mix orange juice with mayonnaise, add apples, celery and raisins to the dressing mixture and stir well.

Serve at room temperature or chilled.

<u>Vegetable Pizza</u> - 1 hour

¾ cup pizza sauce
1 cup broccoli, chopped
1 cup carrots, shredded
½ cup bell pepper, sliced
1 cup reduced fat mozzarella cheese, grated

Preheat oven to 450, Prepare favorite yeast based pizza dough as directed and place on baking sheet. Spoon pizza sauce on pizza shell.

Arrange vegetables over sauce. sprinkle on cheese. Bake for 10 minutes.

When baked, cool pizza for 3 minutes before slicing.

Cut into 8 wedges. Enjoy!

<u>Mixed Steamed Greens</u>

2 bundles of kale
2 bundles of collards 1 small leek
1 teaspoon olive oil sea salt to taste

Put water in a steamer, just below the steamer basket and bring to rapid boil. Wash greens thoroughly. Roll leaves and cut. Place in steamer basket, add salt (optional) and let steam for 5-8 minutes. Remove from basket, place in bowl and add olive oil. Enjoy!

10 Minute Roasted Asparagus

1 pound asparagus
tablespoons extra virgin olive
oil kosher salt or sea salt
freshly ground black pepper
fresh lemon juice (optional)

Heat oven to 450.

Wash asparagus in a colander under cold running water. Cut or snap off the tough woody ends of the asparagus. Discard the ends or save them to use for broth or sauce. Peel the stalks, if desired. Leave the spears whole or cut into shorter lengths. Pat the asparagus dry with paper towels. Toss asparagus spears with 2 tablespoons of olive oil. Arrange the spears in a single layer in the baking pan. Sprinkle lightly with kosher salt or sea salt. Roast for 8 to 10 minutes - tips should appear lightly browned. If desired, sprinkle with black pepper and lemon before serving.

Steamed Root Vegetables

2 small parsnips
1 sweet potato
2 small carrots
1 small rutabaga
1 medium turnip
1 leek
1 tablespoon safflower oil
sea salt to taste

Put water in steamer just below basket and bring to rapid boil. Wash peel and dice all roots and leek. Put in steamer basket add salt and let steam for 10 to 12 minutes.

Remove from steam and place in bowl stir in safflower oil. Serve warm.

Iron

Iron is found in every cell of the body. Iron is important in the diet because it has a central role in supplying oxygen to the body. Iron helps to build and maintain healthy blood. Iron and Iron fortified food serve as deterrents to lead entering the bloodstream. Iron deficiency can be an entryway for lead. Iron deficiency not only weakens the mother but also renders the child helpless to fight off the onslaught of lead contamination. Many expectant women are given iron supplements. Iron strengthens the blood. Some foods that are high in iron are dried beans; iron fortified cereal, dried fruit, and dark green leafy vegetables. Children and women of childbearing age should pay particular attention to receiving enough iron in their diet each day. The following foods are good sources of iron:

Dried Apricots	Beet Greens
Dries Beans or Peas	Dates
Iron Fortified Cereal	Dried Peaches
Sardines	Strawberries

Wheat Germ	Dried Prunes / Prune Juice
Swiss Chard	Eggs
Raisins	Spinach
Tomato Juice	Whole Grain Breads

Lead

Lead is a toxic metal that finds itself into the human body and accumulates in the brain, central nervous system, bones, glands and hair. Lead poisoning can eventually lead to paralysis of the extremities, blindness, mental disturbances, loss of memory, mental retardation and even insanity.

Since the beginning of the industrial revolution, over 60 billion tons of lead has been added to the North American supply. Although vehicle emissions from lead were markedly reduced in 1986, an estimated 4 to 5 million metric tons of lead has accumulated in the soil due to the use of leaded gasoline in previous years.

The most common form or lead exposure and the resulting toxicity are through the ingestion of lead-containing paint, often used in older houses. Ingestion is the primary route of exposure in children.

LEAD IS EVERYWHERE.

It gets in the air through industrial emissions, paint dust, and the burning of solid wastes. Industry and paint chips contaminate the soil with lead. When crops are grown in soil containing lead, the food supply becomes poisoned, is oftentimes not tested and sold anyway. Food can also be contaminated through use of lead-glazed pottery, leaded crystal and food sold in cans soldered with lead. Although the United States has banned the use of lead-soldered cans some imported foods are still sold this way. The United States has also banned the sale of leaded gasoline and lead in plumbing. Still the drinking water in some (older) homes becomes contaminated through the lead solder in water pipes. The runoff from leaded soil can also contaminate groundwater. (Blacks and other so-called minorities are at particular risk of lead poisoning as these groups are more likely to live near highways or industry where emission of lead fumes is common.) Lead is all around us. The key is learning to live safely with lead because lead is going to be around for years to come. While living with lead may be unavoidable children do not have to continue to become poisoned by lead. Lead poisoning is totally preventable.

Major Lead Sources

Paint chips
Lead-based paint
Tobacco smoke Electric cable covering
Dust in and around homes and buildings
Solder
Leaded glass Leaded gasoline
Parental occupations and hobbies
Pottery/ceramic glazes
Newsprint
Dyes
Lead soldered plumbing
Lead acid batteries used in automobiles
Hair coloring agents and other cosmetics
Black and colored inks
Ashes and fumes from burning oil painted wood
Soil and air in and around industrialized areas
Drinking water
Sewage sludge
Waste incineration
Landfills
Food in lead-soldered cans
Liver
Some domestic and imported wines
Insecticides

The following **_Gray Lives Matter_** is an excerpt from the sequel to A Child is a Terrible Thing to Waste.

Gray Lives Matter

What is the Matter?   The Matter is Lead!

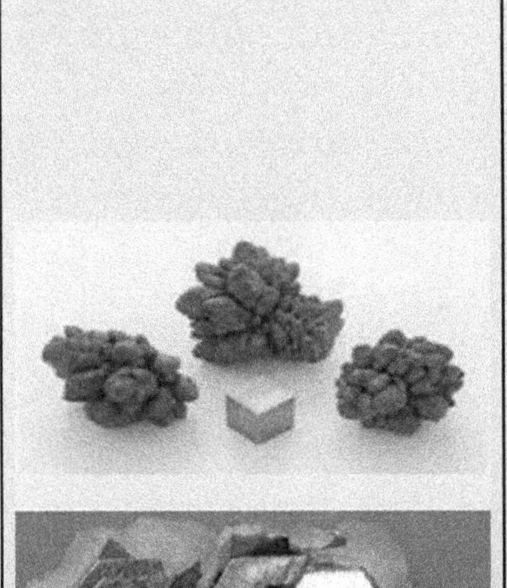

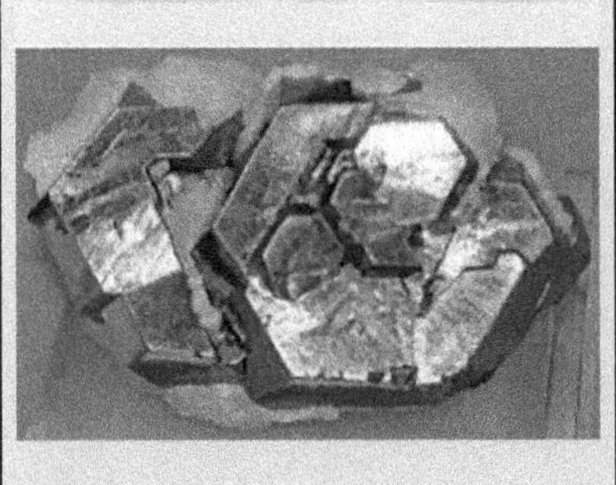

Lead is a chemical element. A heavy metal that is denser than most common materials. Lead is soft and malleable, and also has a relatively low melting point. When freshly cut, lead is silvery with a hint of blue; it tarnishes to a dull gray color when exposed to air.

Symbol: Pb

Atomic number: 82

Did you know: Lead and mercury

Considered as one of the main causes of autism.

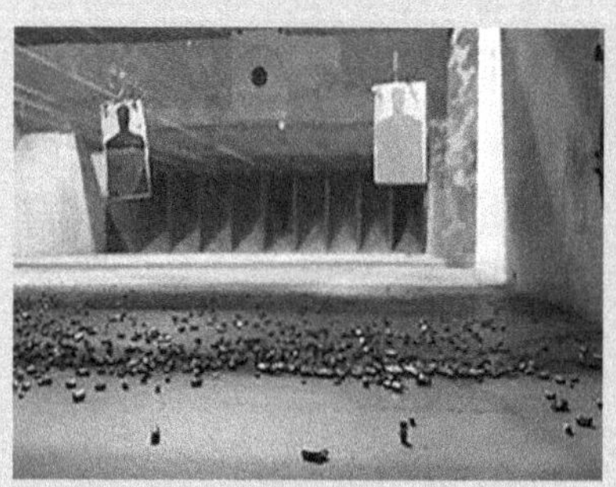

Shooting range - notice the Black and Brownish silhouettes used for target practice. Lead poisoning increases violence - surely police officers are exhibiting extreme displays of violent aggression especially in communities of color.

EACH TIME A BULLET PIERCES A BODY, THAT'S LEAD POISONING

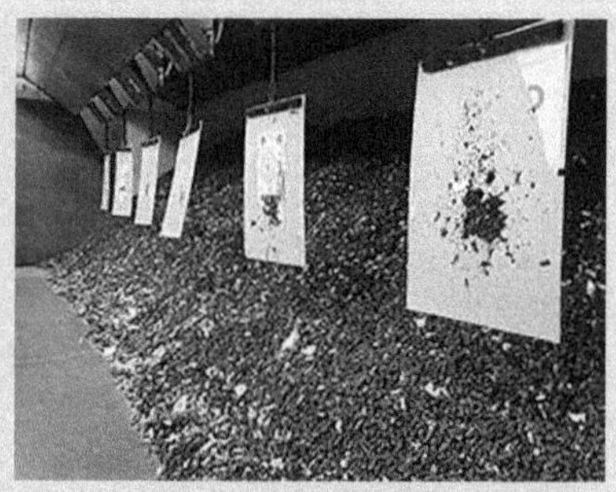

Spent Ammunition - a mass of gray leaded matter - This is of particular interest to me in the fight to have all law enforcement officers have mandatory periodic lead testing, given the enormous rate of innocent and unarmed people of color being shot and killed by police officers. This is an Environmental Justice Issue!

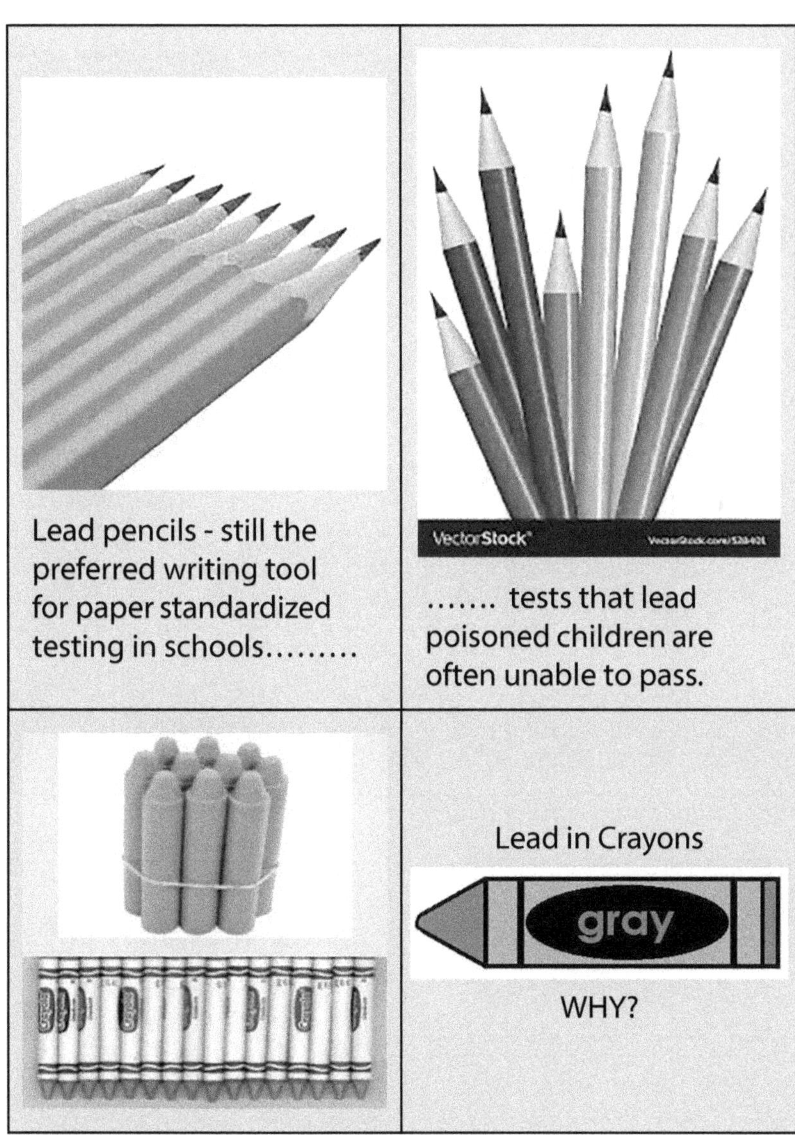

VectorStock®
Lead pencils - still the preferred writing tool for paper standardized testing in schools.........
.... tests that lead poisoned children are often unable to pass.
Lead in Crayons
gray
WHY?

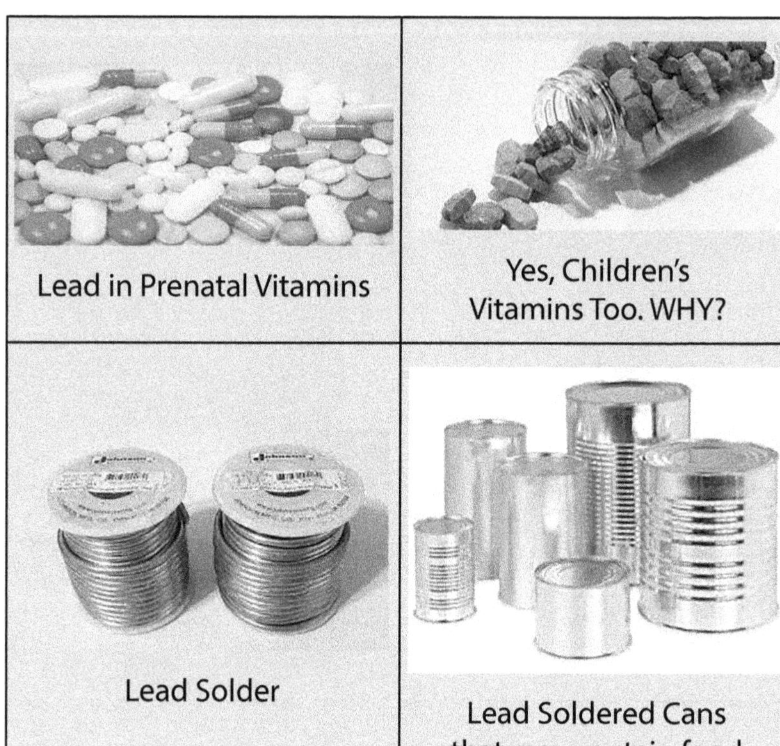
Lead in Prenatal Vitamins
Yes, Children's
Vitamins Too. WHY?
Lead Solder
Lead Soldered Cans
that may contain food

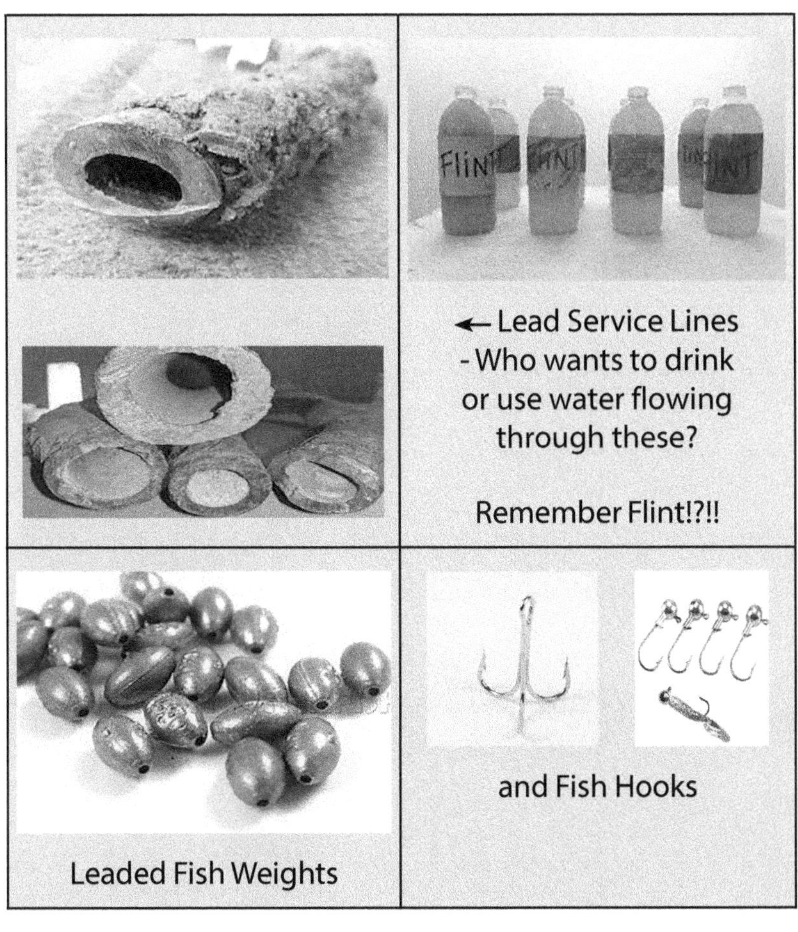

← Lead Service Lines
- Who wants to drink
or use water flowing
through these?

Remember Flint!?!!

and Fish Hooks

Leaded Fish Weights

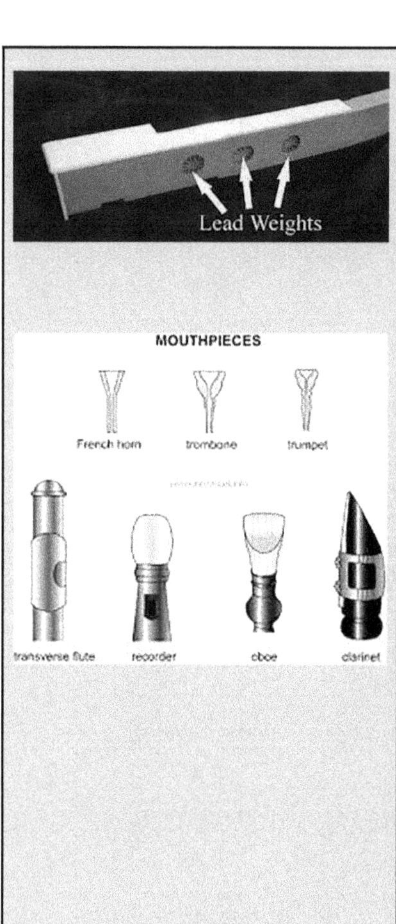

Who Knew?

Lead Found in Brass Mouthpieces Used in Musical Instruments

Center for Env. Health has found the toxic metal lead in 13 brass mouthpieces used to play instruments like trumpets, saxophones, and trombones. CEH sent legal notices to 12 manufacturers and two retailers for failing to warn customers of this health threat, as required by California's consumer protection law Prop 65. Prop 65 identifies lead as a metal that causes cancer and reproductive harm.

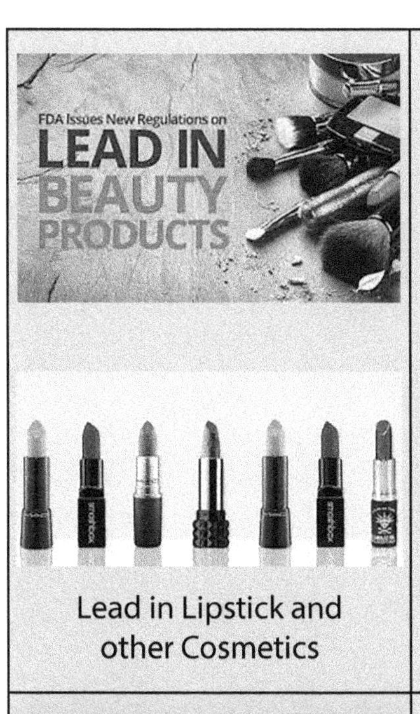

Lead in Lipstick and
other Cosmetics

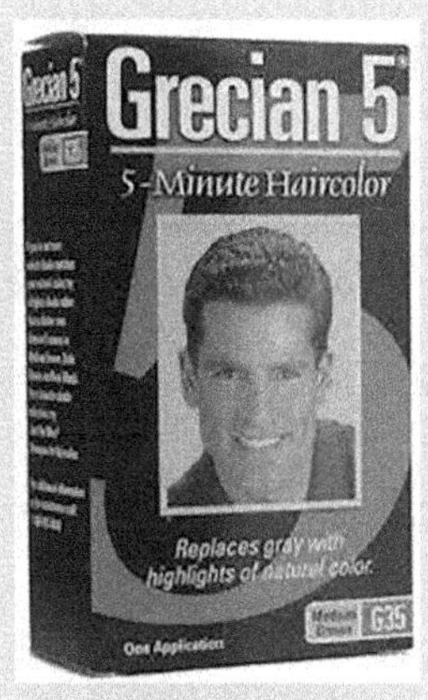

Lead in Hair Dyes 5-
minute poisoning

Using gray to get
rid of the gray

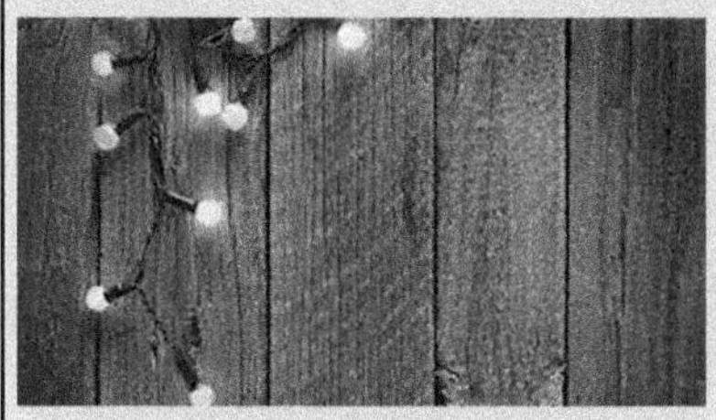

Vinyl Coating on
Christmas Lighting

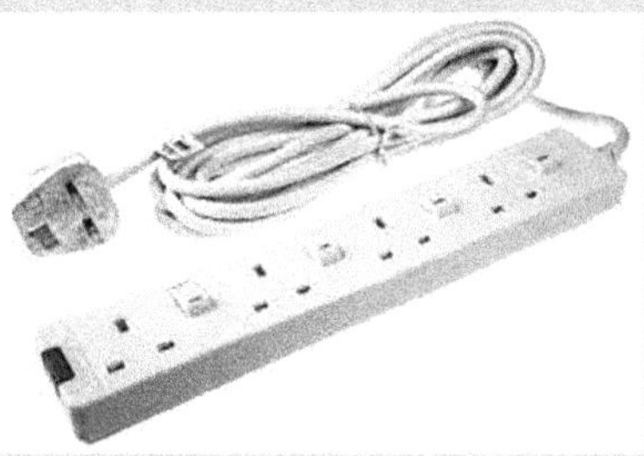

and Extension Cords

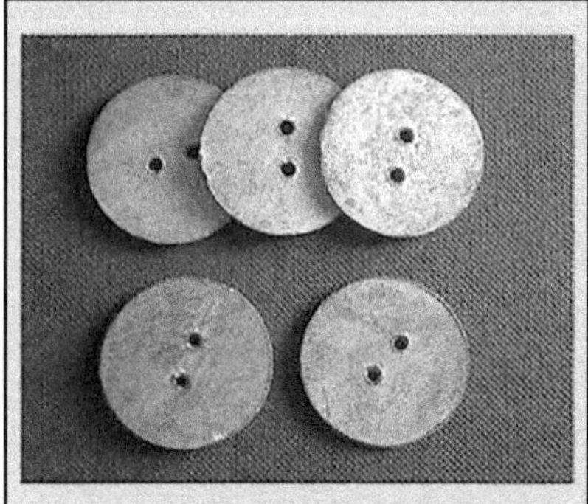

Leaded Penny Weights
used in Curtain Hems

**CHILDREN HAVE BEEN
POISONED BY THESE**

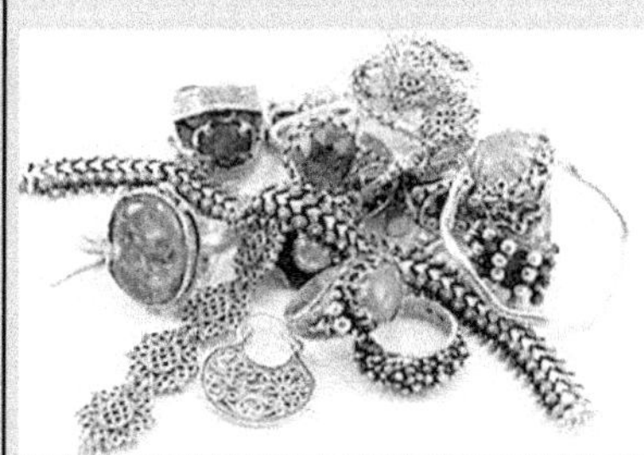

Lead in Jewelry

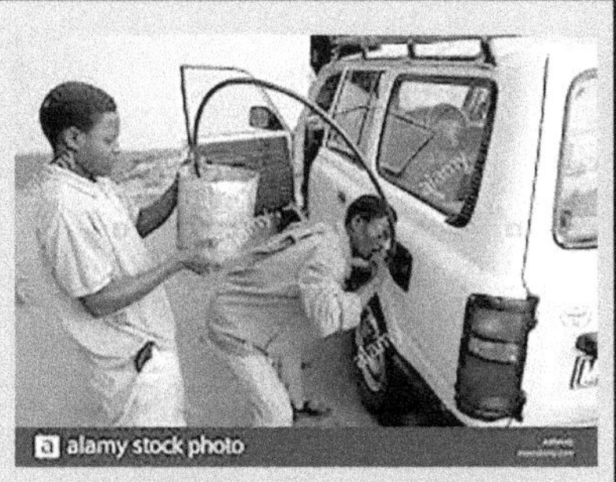

Siphoning Leaded Gasoline to transfer from one vehicle to another. This was a common practice on farms

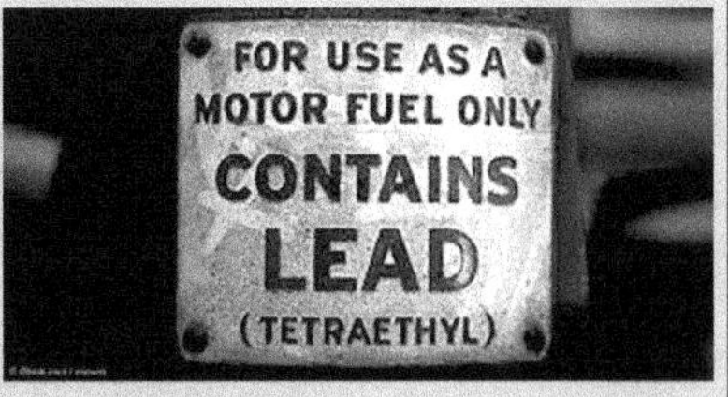

Tetraethyl Lead used to be an additive in gasoline to prevent the dreaded knocking.

Never mind that it permanently harmed people in the process.

Lead Wheel Weights still used on automobiles →

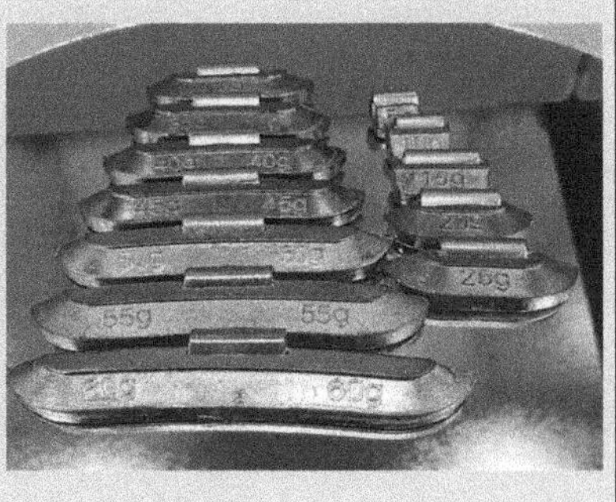

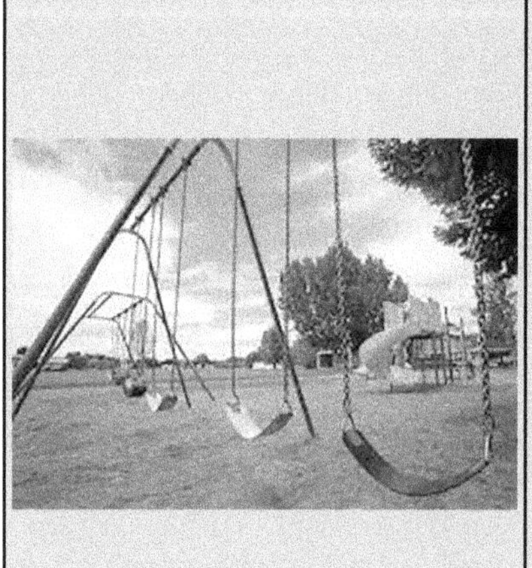

Because of weathering and time, **lead** paint on outdoor **playground equipment** can deteriorate into chips and dust that contain **lead**. Children ingest **lead** paint chips and dust by putting their hands on the **equipment** then placing their hands in their mouths.

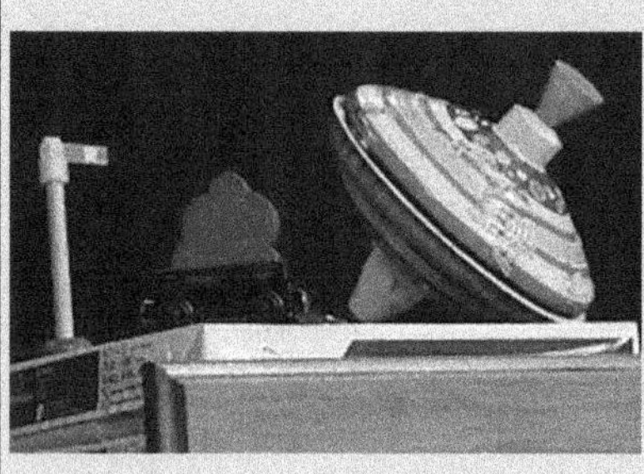

Lead in Children's Toys

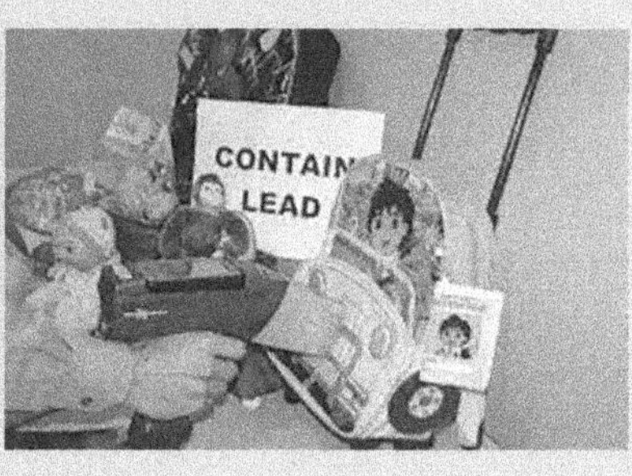

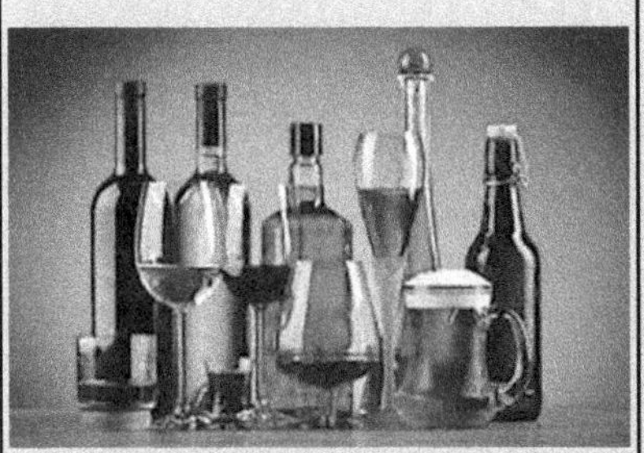

LEAD in Fancy
Wine Bottles

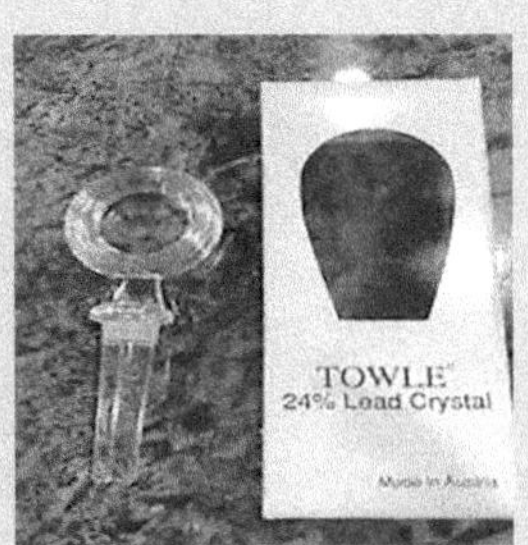

and dainty Crystals

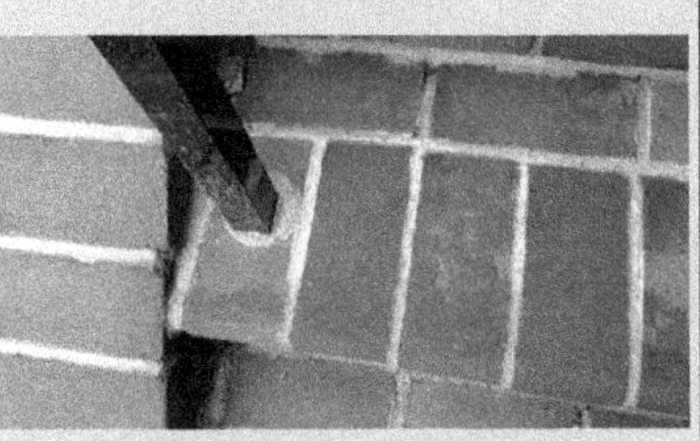

Lead solder around
the banister posts
on the steps at UR

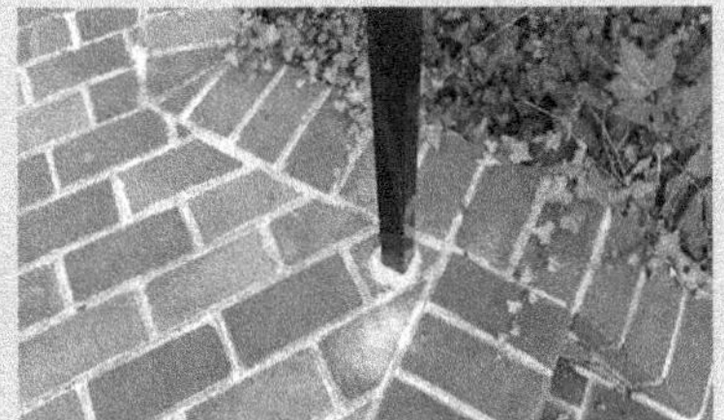

These steps lead to
the Boatwright

Memorial Library and,
like vinyl siding, "should
be generally safe as long
as you don't spend time
licking it or touching it"!

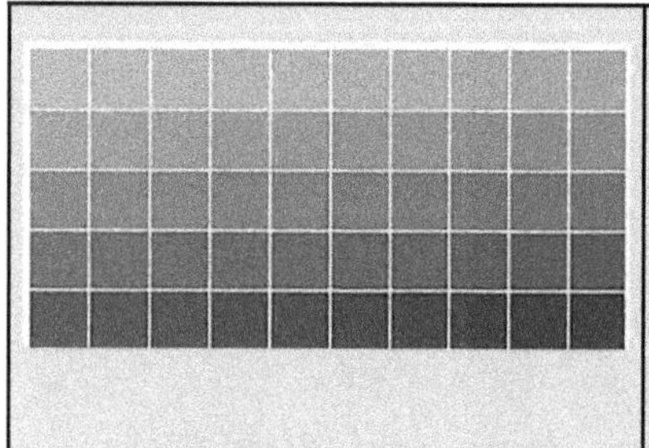

LEAD POISONING CAUSES PERMANENT AND IRREVERSIBLE BRAIN DAMAGE

Protect Children from Lead Poisoning

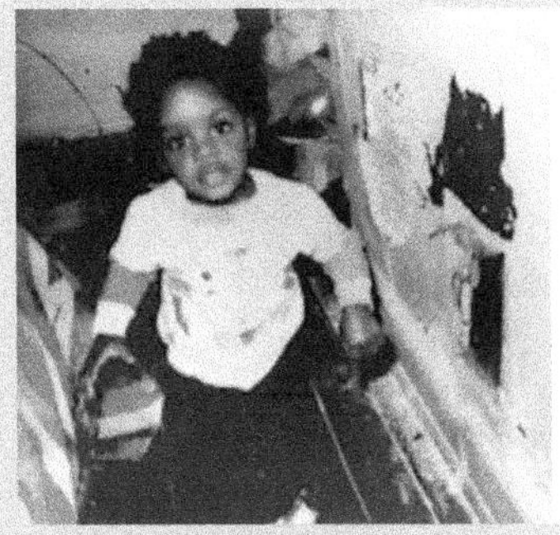
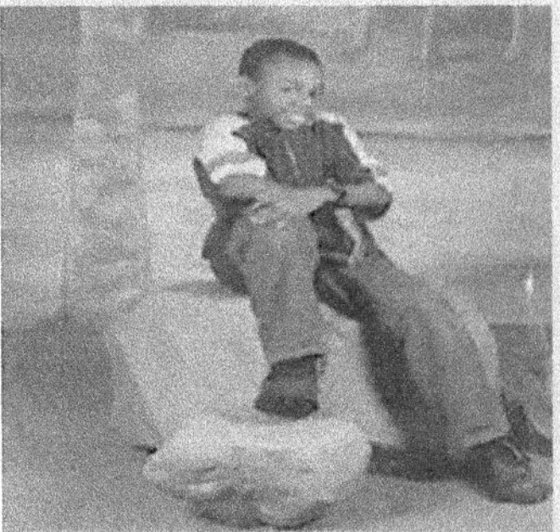

Harm Caused by LEAD Persists a Lifetime

A Young Freddie Gray   A Young Sergio Gray

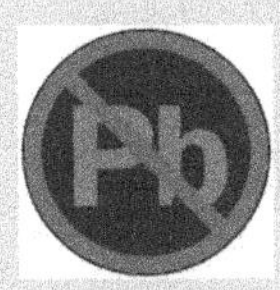

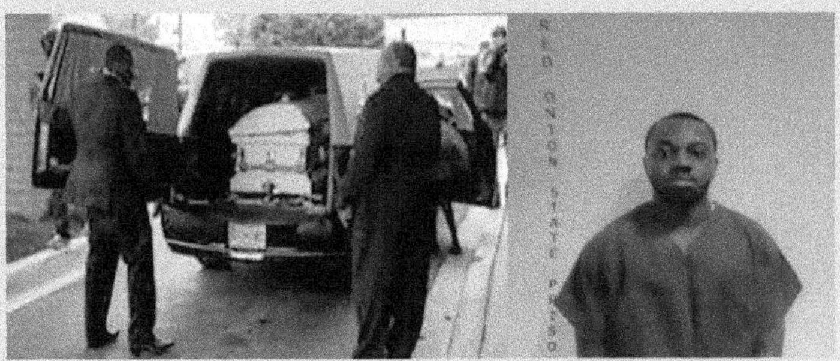

Freddie's Last Ride in   Sergio at Red Onion -
a Silver/Gray Casket   Enough to Make me Cry
                              Now behind the gray
                              walls of Greensville
                              Correctional Center
                              in Jarratt, Virginia.

Chapter 2

Drinking Water - Is It Safe?

Water ranks second to oxygen on the list of substances essential to life. I'm not sure if two bodies were actually tested to determine this but I've read that humans can survive at least a week without consuming food but will succumb only after a few days without water. Water, as much as it is needed, can pose serious threats to those whose lives it sustains.

Is it safe to drink the water? That is a question often pondered and a lot of parents don't know where or who to look to for answers.

You will not be able to see, smell or taste lead in your water. Testing is the only way to be sure. Your local health department or the Environmental Protection Agency (EPA) can recommend a state-certified testing lab. Preliminary steps to take include inspecting your plumbing and talking with your water utility company. The water utility company should be able to tell you whether the system or service connections contain lead. Lead is a dull gray metal that is easily scratched.

This is what you should look for when inspecting your plumbing. Pay particular attention to the pipes where they join.

Pipes made before 1930 are most likely solid lead while some brass fixtures may also contain lead.

Know your water type. Some water is referred to as "soft." Soft water is acidic and eats away at plumbing. Lead from the pipes then dissolves into the water and is delivered to your family through your tap. One way to protect your family is by flushing your plumbing. This is done by letting the cold water run a while before using it for drinking or cooking.

You should always flush your plumbing if it has not been used for six hours or more, especially overnight. Be sure to use cold water because hot water causes more pipe corrosion and will have higher levels of lead. If you can afford to, you can have your plumbing replaced with lead-free materials or use a water treatment system that specifically states that it removes lead.

Amendments and new regulations to The Safe Drinking Water Act of 1974 have banned the use of lead in new plumbing and plumbing repairs. There has also been a reduction in permissible lead levels in drinking water. A 1988 amendment included testing school water to prevent lead contamination.

Bottled water and water-softening agents should not be relied upon entirely in efforts to avoid lead poisoning. Bottled water may contain as much as is allowed in household tap water. Water softeners are designed to remove calcium and magnesium. They are not designed to remove lead.

I urge you to use whatever method feasible to protect your family from lead and other water contaminants. Make sure your drinking water is safe.

For more information contact EPA's Safe Drinking Water Information Hotline: 1-800.426.4791.

Book II:

My Family's Battle With Pb

We can do little

against an invisible

or unknown enemy.

Chapter 3

Methods of Testing for Lead

Most lead poisoning cases go undiagnosed because there are no obvious symptoms. As parents you are urged to have your children tested. Prevention and early detection are key to ensuring that children live up to their full potential.

Common methods of testing:

1. **The finger prick** - as it implies a child's fingertip is pricked and a small sample of blood tested. This method is not highly recommended as it may show a false positive if the child has recently been exposed to a leaded object or surface.

2. **Venous blood test** - with this method blood is drawn directly from a vein in the child's arm. This method is preferable, more reliable and highly recommended. Blood tests will reveal only the most recent exposure.

3. **Hair analysis** - hair clippings are sent to a certified lab to detect the lead levels. This method is commonly used to accurately determine past exposure and long-term accumulation of lead.

4. **Bone analysis** – this method is also used to determine the number of years exposed.

5. **Teeth analysis** - tests for lead content In teeth.

Tooth lead analysis

The American Association for Clinical Chemistry publication: Directory of Rare Analyses, indicates that National Medical Services (NMS), performs lead testing in Hair, Nails and other specimens for post-mortem or forensic cases. NMS also offers tooth lead testing as a "Special Request" test. They do not however work with private individuals. A person would need to either go through a Dr., Lawyer or another lab in order for NMS to do the testing.

National Medical Services (NMS), 2300 Stratford Avenue, Willow Grove, PA, 19090-4195 USA
PH: 2156574900 or free call USA 800-522-6671
EMAIL: nms@nmslab.com WEB: www.nmslab.com

This was of utmost importance to me because Zaki's teeth suffered the most damage in his bout with lead.

For additional information call National Medical Services at 215.657.4900.

The Centers for Disease Control (CDC) has set the minimum lead level of concern at 5 micrograms per deciliter in blood (5 ug/dL). Again, blood tests will only reveal recent or continued exposure to lead.

There are various Home lead testing kits on the market that allow you to test for lead in water, paint, glass, ceramics, soil and dust. These kits can be found in hardware and home product stores.

There are a series of questions that are designed to determine if your child is at "high risk" for lead exposure. If you answer yes to any one of the following questions you should have your child tested for lead poisoning.

1. Does your child live in a pre-1960 house with peeling, chipping, and flaking lead based-paint? (consider also whether this description applies to your daycare, baby-sitters or often visited relative's homes)

2. Does your child live in or regularly visit a house that's undergoing remodeling or renovation?

3. Does your child live with an adult who is exposed to lead in his/her workplace? Occupations include home renovation workers or contractors, employees in battery factories, recycling plants or lead smelters.

   (These adults may be bringing home lead dust on their clothing*).

4. Does your child live near a battery factory, battery recycling plant or lead smelter? There is a high possibility that the entire neighborhood is contaminated.

5. Does your child have a sibling or playmate who's currently being tested for lead poisoning?

I think it is safe and wise to have all children tested whether or not you answered yes to any of the above questions. Even children who appear healthy can have dangerous levels of lead. Lead is more dangerous to children than adults because their growing bodies absorb more lead. Their brains and central nervous systems are developing and more sensitive to the damaging effects of lead.

*Although it is common to hear more about childhood lead poisoning there are many adults who also suffer from over exposure to lead. I urge adults to have themselves tested as well and take all precautions to avoid contact with this deadly metal.

Adults with high levels of lead may suffer from reproductive problems (men and women), high blood pressure, digestive problems, nerve disorders, memory and concentration problems and muscle and joint pain. Note also that smokers have significantly higher lead levels than non smokers and previous smokers.

Chapter 4

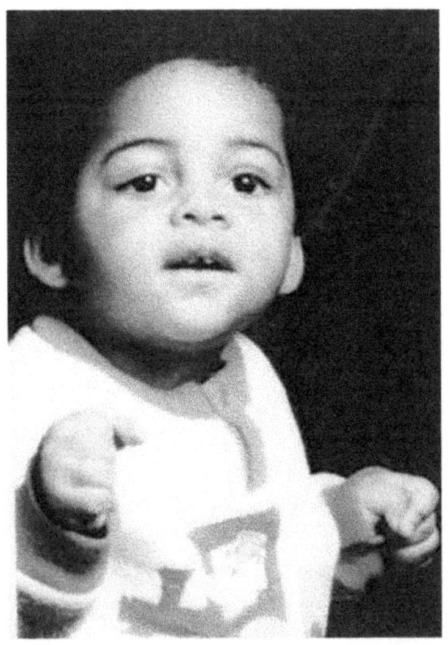

ZAKI

Zaki was born with balled fists.
I knew he would be a fighter

"The world when seen through

a little child's eyes,

greatly resembles paradise."

Those glimpses of paradise can be dimmed or nullified once a child is poisoned by lead. My son Zaki's paradise was almost stolen by lead. As a mother I vowed to fight back with everything I had in me against this silent enemy. When Zaki was stricken we as a family banded together to give him and each other the strength and support we all needed to survive the unwelcome intrusion.

Venous 30. (venous is one of the many words added to my vocabulary that I would now use in regular everyday conversation). That was Zaki's initial blood lead level when he was first tested in February of 1996. One week later his lead level had dropped to 18. With one simple test our family was hurled into a new world. Lead poisoning is a world unto itself. We had no idea that all of the new terms and definitions would become such an intricate part of all of our lives. Zaki became our focus. We were all concerned and wanted to save him. We were all worried that he had sustained some damages that no one but the Supreme Being would be able to repair. Zaki was poisoned but why, where and how did he get that way?

I had not even thought about lead poisoning for years. If I did read any articles about it, they were vaguely remembered or altogether dismissed. For lead was of no consequence to me. Lead had no part, no connection in my life. It has been said that the mind is like a computer (or is it that computers are fashioned after the mind?). I don't even know why I thought of lead poisoning when I saw the peeling, chipping paint that was around the window air conditioning unit in my children's room. Something clicked and the memories of my cousin Tony came flooding back. I immediately called our pediatrician and arranged to have all four of my children tested. Luckily for Zaki, Dr. Carolyn Boone is one of the few pediatricians in Richmond who will screen for lead without the parent having to do everything short of getting a court order.

The CDC had established, at that time, that a child having a blood lead level equal or greater than 10 ug/dL (micrograms per deciliter, another term that has become common to me) is a lead poisoned child. Zaki's level of 30 was very frightening. Even more frightening was the fact that he had shown absolutely no signs of being ill. Had he not been tested he would have continued being exposed to lead and because we would not have known what precautions to take to protect him, his lead level could have gotten even higher.

Dr. Boone notified the local health department of Zaki's elevated blood lead level. Now the real drama begins. I was filled with so many questions that I couldn't get them out fast enough. The answers were not always to my satisfaction but I kept asking anyway. I was blessed to meet some really wonderful people who are lead poisoning prevention advocates and who I probably never would have met if my son was not poisoned. So it is true that some good always comes out of the bad. Still there were subtle hints from time to time that I must have been less than a good mother and my house cleaning skills must have been below par for my son to have been poisoned. Although as a Black woman domesticity is in my genes and I couldn't get away from it if I try and I have tried occasionally. So yes, the fingers were pointed at me, as they are pointed at most parents of lead poisoned children. We are asked stupid questions like "Did you see her eating paint chips?" and "So you allowed him to play in the dirt?" As if you were out of corn flakes one morning so instead you sat a bowl of paint chips in front of the child. And what mother in her right mind would intentionally tell her child not to play on the green grass but play over there in the leaded dirt where the grass won't grow? There was even a lawsuit in Virginia in which the defense attorneys tried unsuccessfully to introduce into court the IQs of the parents of a lead poisoned child. The attorney's premise was that the child did not have learning disabilities because of lead poisoning but was just born dumb because the parents were dumb. The judge in this case decided wisely not to admit this line of questioning. Some of the healthcare workers that I came in contact with, while they may be good administratively and medically, they have no people skills. It is already hard enough for parents to deal with the news that their child is poisoned but to have to be accused of somehow inflicting this upon your child is double jeopardy. So I've had to exchange harsh words with some and have had a few scrimmages along the way but it has been worth the effort to see my son overcome, thrive and survive. The few run-ins I've had with health care workers in Richmond are nothing in comparison to some of the horror stories I've heard from my state counterparts. Indeed, I must say that staff members of the local and state health departments, Lead-Safe Richmond and Virginia Department of Health's (VDH) Lead-Safe Virginia Childhood Lead Poisoning Prevention programs have both been very supportive of me, my family and the UPAL of Virginia Chapter. They encouraged and provided technical support for the programs that UPAL has implemented and proffered monetary assistance as well. At times they even offer moral support, which is not always easy, because it is sometimes difficult to understand what a mother is feeling if you yourself are not the parent of a lead poisoned child. Yet they have been there to show compassion and understanding even during the times when I may have been difficult to get along with. For this I am appreciative and forever thankful.

Zaki was only 21 months old when he was diagnosed. Like most children he showed absolutely no signs of being poisoned. I was in tears after receiving the call that he had an elevated blood lead level. Zaki was then the youngest of six children so he was the baby to all of us. Although I was not yet educated on the various degrees of lead poisoning I knew that 30 was not good. I had no idea what this meant to my son's future. It was then that I decided to become proactive. I had no idea what to do or where to start but I knew I had to do something. I talked to anyone who would talk to me. I asked many, many questions. I was determined to save my child and eventually this quest would grow to envelop all children. I got so involved and engulfed by the issues of lead poisoning that other parts of my life were left unattended and suffered. My husband and I would eventually divorce after 18 years of marriage.

Sometimes when you get bad news you become traumatized and immobilized. Although we took immediate action to reduce Zaki's exposure and his lead level dropped significantly within one week he didn't escape damage entirely. Zaki's teeth were worst hit. Lead competes with calcium. Calcium deficiencies can enhance the effects of lead. Dentists would tell me that it was because of his sucking a baby bottle. For me, as a parent, to suggest that he had acquired tooth decay as a result of being poisoned by lead one would think that I had somehow insulted their ability as a dentist. So after I'd heard them out about the baby bottle, I would triumphantly say "but he never drank from a bottle he was totally breast fed," as were all of my children. The dentist would then start stuttering and some looked at me like I had to be lying. Any way I kept searching until I found one (a pediatric dentist Dr. Arthur Mourino at the Medical College of Virginia's School of Dentistry) who at least acknowledged that it is possible. I mentioned to him that I had found a lab that would test the teeth for lead content and he was anxious to know the results too.

Zaki has had to have all of his upper front teeth extracted. Six teeth all at the same time. He has endured like a champ. He is still quick to smile and it certainly has not stopped him from talking as much. When Zaki was last tested on July 26, 1999 his blood lead level had dropped from 5 to 3. He will be tested again in one year. Our goal is that his results will be "0."

It is any parent's worst nightmare to have their child hurt and not be able to protect them. To a mother who had buried a son, the news of Zaki's lead poisoning was devastating. Zaki's oldest brother, Shaheen was laid to rest at the tender age of seven. He succumbed to congestive heart failure. I held him in my arms as he took his last breath. Helpless to do anything to help him, save him, relieve him from the obvious pain, bring him back. At that moment I felt overwhelmingly powerless. So naturally when Zaki was diagnosed with lead poisoning I found it difficult to breathe. Since burying my first-born son, I became overprotective of my other children. Always fearful that something might happen to them, I didn't let them out of my sight. I even home schooled them for many years. I kept them at home locked in with a hazard unbeknown to me. We locked the doors every night and still the enemy got in. Was actually there waiting for us when we moved in. The city of Richmond assisted my family in moving into the house that endangered my children. Officials were aware of my children's ages yet no one mentioned to us the danger of lead poisoning. No one suggested that the house be tested. Not a word about lead. Not a word until it was too late. Everyone got moving and was ready to act AFTER THE FACT. It angered me so that most of the time I was unsure exactly what emotions I was feeling. I was scared for Zaki, mad at the city, mad at the health department, detested the house, Frantic! Afraid that death would come visiting again I prayed {Oh Lord don't take me son.} I knew my heart could not bear to see another child of mine buried.

When my prayers were answered and I found that there was something I could do about the alien that had invaded my child's body I made a vow to him that I would not rest until his body was free of lead.

We can do little against an unknown or invisible enemy, but when parents know that someone or something specific is threatening the wellbeing of their most prized possessions they will fight and do whatever it takes to be victorious. So when the enemy was identified and given a name and a history, the battle was on. The lioness in me was unleashed. My cubs had been threatened. My baby cub had been injured. This thing called Lead was going to pay.

As I readied myself for the battle, gathering ammunition and studying lead's historical tactics I was filled with a force that was equally as powerful as the helplessness I had felt at the death of my son Shaheen. At that moment I knew that lead would be defeated. I knew I was in for a battle but I had no idea of the magnitude of the war.

Book III

The Cure

No drug can cure disease. Lasting results can only be attained when a wise doctor educates his patient and then both work to assist and support the body's own healing forces until health is accomplished.

- Hippocrates

Chapter 5

Treatment for Lead Toxicity

My first priority was to get the lead out of Zaki's system. Zaki's exposure was caught in time to prevent any further damage that might have happened. As I said previously his lead level dropped from 30 to 18 in one week. Six months later it was down to 12.

In one year after the initial diagnosis Zaki's lead level had dropped to 5 where it held steady until July 1999. While I am pleased that his level steadily declined and did not yo-yo I still strive for a level of zero. This is how we treated Zaki:

After giving him a (weak strength) cleansing herbal tea for three days, I immediately increased Zaki's consumption of fiber, beans (dried), fruits rich in Vitamin-C (kiwi, strawberries, lemons, oranges,) and seaweed products.

These foods contain compounds that bind to heavy metals and help the body to excrete them. These effective lead binders are known as "chelators." We avoided tap water and drank steam-distilled water instead, to which I sometimes add aloe vera juice. I also fed Zaki more eggs, onions and garlic. While there is no common approach for the treatment of lead toxicity at present health and nutritional counseling is probably the most cost effective means to use with children whose exposure is less than 20 ug/dL. Children whose level are higher than 20 should receive more involved intervention. Possible treatment might include reducing the child's body burden and absorption of lead, chelation therapy, treating calcium and iron deficiency and removing sources of lead. Whenever possible, REMOVE THE CHILD FROM THE LEADED ENVIRONMENT.

Zaki's lead level was not high enough to necessitate his hospitalization, and since his level rapidly declined in a matter of days, I decided to stick with natural remedies and avoid all medications. Following are some methods that I came across in my search.

Uropathy

Uropathy is Urine Therapy. During my research I came across a book written by Martin J. Lara in which he describes the natural treatment of drinking one's own urine. While I am not advocating that anyone practice Uropathy I did note that the book contained a section on lead poisoning and that got my attention. I also do not condemn those who are brave and open minded enough to try it. The following "recipes" are reprinted with permission from Martin Lara's book Uropathy:

1. Fast for 30 days on water and urine only.

2. Rub or massage the whole body or the affected area with two to eight-day-old urine. Rinse it off with cool water after 15 minutes. Do not use soap.

3. Drink one to four ounces of fresh urine in the morning. The urine can be pure or mixed with juice.

Vitamin C

According to the September, 1998 issue of "Healthy Universe" published by the Wellness Council of America: VITAMIN C Gets the Lead Out. In a recent study, men who took 1,000 mg of vitamin c every day lowered their blood lead levels dramatically in just one week. Lead detoxification may be helpful for restoring male fertility in some cases.

Oral Chelation

There is a company called Extreme Health, Inc. that claims to have a "revolutionary" product that "excreted 350% lead from 14 patients after just one day of use". The product is called Oral Chelation and Ageless Formula and touted as being a "Powerful All Natural Formula" that will "Help Reverse & Prevent Mercury, Lead and other Heavy Metal Toxicity". The Oral Chelation and the Ageless Formula come in two vitamin-like containers of 60 capsules each. I have spoken extensively with a representative of the company who sent me samples of the formula. She stated that the formula is "a natural, plant based formula that binds to heavy metal and replenishes where there was damage caused by metals. It also supports the kidney and liver." The formula has no FDA approval because it is "like a vitamin." Years after "A Child is a Terrible to Waste" was first published we found that LEAD was also an ingredient in some children's vitamins.

*I do not recommend or endorse these products for use. I myself do not use them although they claim to be "all natural." I mention them here only for your knowledge and awareness of what is available. I have received writings on these two products but have not ascertained their safety, contents, FDA approval, (which may or may not mean anything good). I understand that there was a single blind study of 20 children aged 5-15 conducted. I do not have the results of that study. I caution you to use at your own risk and be aware that our children, who have suffered lead poisoning and the many ills associated with it, are always prone to be used as guinea pigs by companies who will seek financial gain because they are able to play on our (the parents') emotions. Beware!

Chapter 6

Garlic

The herb called Garlic has long been touted as one of the world's oldest medicines.

European studies have shown that garlic helps eliminate lead and other toxic heavy metals from the body. In my search to find natural remedies to rid Zaki's body of lead contamination garlic was the most mentioned Garlic grows all over the world and has literally hundreds of healing uses ranging from treating tonsillitis and infections to lowering cholesterol levels to combating life threatening diseases. Garlic, nature's miracle plant, has a powerful history. It was used 6,000 years ago to increase strength and endurance and for its healing properties. The ancient Egyptians fed garlic to the laborers who built the great pyramids. Later the Greeks and the Romans were reported to have consumed garlic in large amounts. Their strength, endurance and resistance to disease were attributed to their garlic consumption.

Hippocrates, the so-called father of medicine, was perhaps actually an herbalist and natural healer. He is said to have used garlic to treat many diseases including cancer.

Garlic, the leading over the counter drug in many Asian and European countries, is a broad-spectrum antibiotic, antiviral agent and fungicide.

Garlic is now being used to treat heart disease, high blood pressure and colon-rectal (as well as other forms of) cancer. As an antibiotic, diluted garlic juice has been found to inhibit the growth of bacteria. Garlic destroys many types of bacteria including streptococcus, staphylococcus, typhoid, diphtheria, cholera, bacterial dysentery (traveler's diarrhea), tuberculosis, tetanus, rheumatic bacteria and even the bacteria that causes leprosy.

I list the many wonders of garlic because again, I prefer natural means and sometimes the medicines that are used to heal us and make us better actually do more harm than good. For instance, pharmaceutical antibiotics are prescribed indiscriminately to the point of gross over use. These antibiotics are non-selective in their destruction of bacteria and attack the millions of friendly bacteria as well. In addition to our bodies becoming immune to these antibiotics many people develop digestive problems, constipation and yeast and fungal infections. Consequently, dangerous resistant strains of bacteria are created and the antibiotics are useless against them. Garlic on the other hand is selective in its destruction of bacteria. While killing only the harmful bacteria it simultaneously enhances our friendly bacteria and improves digestion.

In our battle against lead poisoning Garlic is what worked for us. That simple clove. Nothing spectacular or new. Garlic. I add it liberally to just about everything we eat. I am convinced the raw garlic helped to speed up Zaki's eradication of lead. One day I just gave him a small sliver of raw garlic and he ate it and asked for more. Maybe in his innocent wisdom he knew that it was good for him. Despite the taste, he ate it without fuss. I gave it to him daily and sure enough his lead level dropped drastically in a matter of weeks. I have no documentation to compare but I have been told that lead can sometimes take years to diminish. I know of some children whose levels linger and were at the same level when I met them two to three years ago. I urge those parents and all parents of lead poisoned children to try garlic. If the child won't eat it raw then cook it in their favorite foods. Just get the garlic into their bodies and watch the lead go away like Dracula.

Book IV:

UNITED PARENTS AGAINST LEAD

United We Can Save a Rainbow of Children

A CHILD IS A TERRIBLE THING TO WASTE!

Chapter 7

A Child Is A Terrible Thing To Waste!

I think the time finally came that I had bugged the local health department Lead- Safe Richmond employees so much that they grew tired of me. In July of 1996 they introduced me to Maurci Jackson. I met Maurci at a statewide conference on lead education during Lead Poisoning Prevention Week.

Maurci is founder of Parents Against Lead and United Parents Against Lead based in Chicago, Illinois. I was so anxious to meet her and when I finally did I bombarded her with questions. We cried silent tears together as we often do now. Before the evening was over I had decided that we would charter an UPAL chapter in the State of Virginia. Maurci was scheduled to fly back to Chicago that night. She mailed the information that we needed to get started and on September 10, 1996, UPAL of Virginia was incorporated! Thanks to the Lead-Safe Richmond office that saw a need for parents to be empowered and organized. They brought Maurci and I together. It is out of their urgency and support that UPAL of Virginia exists today. The Virginia Chapter became the 13Th UPAL chapter. For more information on UPAL National visit our website at: UPAL (upalnational.org)

In 1997 Maurci Jackson named me Co Executive Director of UPAL National. We have now added our 18Th Chapter and are planning a national conference in the year 2000. The conference will be hosted in Richmond, Virginia, in April, "Lead Awareness Month."

While many milestones have been made there is still much work to be done. I am particularly concerned with the funds going towards so many studies. Some of which you never, ever hear of the outcome. I have attended many meetings and many notes were taken and committees were established and then months will go by without a word. For instance, I have been "appointed" to the (senate/house) joint subcommittee "studying" lead poisoning prevention. I was advised of this appointment in a letter dated June 21, 1999. As of October 8, 1999 no meetings have been set and I have heard no more regarding this study. I for one have grown weary of all of the studying. I think that efforts and funding should go towards sharing the information that is known about lead poisoning and prevention with the public. The masses are still not receiving the necessary basic information. Lead poisoning is always swept under the rug and given second priority when something else comes along. No there is nothing glamorous about lead but it does exist. It is a daily reality. My Leader, Teacher and Guide, The Most Honorable Elijah Muhammad used to say, "delayed justice is denied justice." I think that by conducting studies on top of studies is a way of delaying and thereby denying justice to those who are most affected. After all those conducting the studies feel as if they have all the time in the world because they most often do not have lead poisoned children. Those who have not walked in our shoes can't know the alarm and helplessness that we feel. When your child is ailing you do not have the luxury of time. When you are seeking answers you do not have time to wait for the results of a lingering study. We need answers now. We need results and remedies now. We need access to accurate information now. While you are studying our children are dying.

A Child is a Terrible Thing to Waste

By Zakia Shabazz

When I hear "Get the Lead out"
The words
Have a different meaning For me
Lead poisoning?
I mean
I've been trying to do just that - get the Lead
Out of my child
And your children too
And you
And to some it's no big deal
But my baby son is ill
And I thought I was dreaming
When
I woke up screaming
MY CHILD!?!
A CHILD
A CHILD and LEAD
IS A TERRIBLE THING
A CHILD IS A TERRIBLE THING TO WASTE!

Written and copyrighted in 1997
By Zakia Shabazz
All Rights Reserved

Chapter 8

Death By Lead

Children Learn What They Live
By Dorothy Law Nolte

"If children live with criticism, They learn to condemn.

If children live with hostility, They learn to fight.

If children live with ridicule, They learn to be shy.

If children live with shame, They learn to feel guilty.

If children live with tolerance, They learn to be patient.

If children live with encouragement, They learn confidence.

If children live with praise, They learn to appreciate.

If children live with fairness, They learn justice.

If children live with security, They learn to have faith.

If children live with approval, They learn to like themselves,

If children live with acceptance and Friendship,

They learn to find love in the world."

If children are poisoned by lead, They may not live!

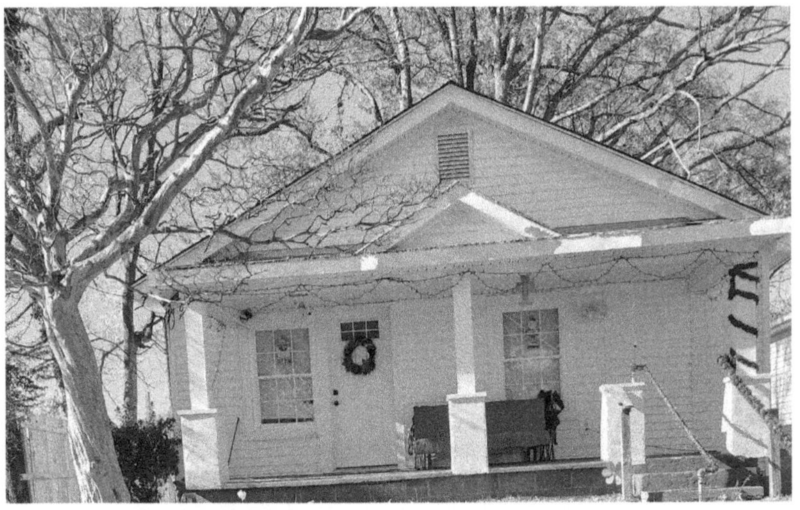

This is the house that poisoned Zaki
1522 East 18th Street, Richmond, VA

This last chapter is dedicated to a 28 month old little boy who lost his life to lead. The year was 1990 in the state of Wisconsin. What you are about to read is excerpted from the Morbidity and Mortality Weekly Report (MMWR) published by the Centers for Disease Control as it appeared in the March 29, 1991 issue. Volume 40 No. 12.

Fatal Pediatric Poisoning

From Leaded Paint - Wisconsin, 1990

Although fatal lead poisoning among children occurs rarely in the United States, it represents a medical and public health emergency. This report summarizes the investigation of a child who died from poisoning associated with ingestion of lead-based paint.

On September 12, 1990, a 28-month-old Wisconsin boy was admitted to a hospital with a 4-day history of lethargy and reduced appetite. Although the child had no known past medical problems, his parents reported that he had eaten flaking paint. On initial neurologic examination, the child had extreme lethargy with facial palsy and gasping respirations, consistent with lead encephalopathy; laboratory results revealed severe lead toxicity and hematologic abnormalities (blood lead level [BLL] 144 ug/dL; erythrocyte protoporphyrin level 593 ug/dL; hemoglobin 8.1; and basophilic stippling.) Despite chelation therapy with British anti Lewisite (Dimercaprol) and calcium disodium edetate (CaNa2-EDTA), the child developed seizures, became comatose, and died within 26 hours after admission. An autopsy showed massive cerebral edema with uncal herniation. The intestines contained multiple roundworms (Ascaris lumbricoides) and flake-like material consistent with paint chips. Radiographs revealed prominent epiphyseal lines in the lower extremities, consistent with chronic lead exposure.

On September 20, staff from the Wisconsin Division of Health and the Waukesha County Health Department inspected the child's residence. The child and his parents had lived for at least 4 months on the second floor of a two story, nonresidential structure built in 1923. The interior paint was badly deteriorated with paint chips visibly flaking from the walls and accumulating on floors, windowsills, and stairs. Eleven paint chip samples from the apartment ranged from 0.2% to 33.1% lead by weight (average 9.1%); the U.S. Consumer Product Safety Commission (CPSC) permits a maximum of 0.06% lead in new residential paint. House dust from the child's bedroom floor contained 3900 ug lead/ft2, and the dust from a windowsill above the child's bed contained 31,128 ug lead/ft2. These levels are more than 10 times higher than those proposed in recent guidelines issued by the U.S. Department of Housing and Urban Development (1), which recommend the maximum dust lead levels permissible before re-occupancy of a unit following lead paint abatement.

After the child's death, the parents moved and were unavailable for follow-up. The landlord had blocked access to the second floor and plans to eliminate the lead paint hazards in the building.

I find this an appropriate way to conclude this book. It is my intention to spark something in you as a reader to become active in preventing this dreadful calamity from claiming the lives of any more children. This child made the ultimate sacrifice. At 28 months he died needlessly. Perhaps by him giving his life and us remembering how and why will save so many others.

Remember the children who have not yet been screened for lead. Remember the 1 million or more children that are presently poisoned. Remember a 28 month-old baby boy in Wisconsin with a blood lead level of **144.** Remember that childhood lead poisoning is totally preventable and A CHILD IS A TERRIBLE THING TO WASTE!!!

State Lead Laws

Less than 20% of counties throughout the US have mandatory lead testing for children. Lead testing is simple and inexpensive to perform.

Below is a brief list of the lead laws in Virginia around 1999. § 54.1-501 Powers and duties of the Board

The Board shall administer and enforce this chapter. The Board shall:

1. Promulgate regulations necessary to carry out the requirements of this chapter in accordance with the provisions of the Administrative Process Act (§9-6.14:1 et seq.) to include but not limited to the prescription of fees, procedures, and qualifications for the issuance and renewal of asbestos and lead licenses, and governing conflicts of interest between various categories of asbestos and lead licenses;

2. Approve the criteria for training courses and primary instructors;

3. Approve training courses, examinations and the grading system for testing applicants for asbestos and lead licensure;

4. Promulgate regulations governing the licensing of and establishing performance criteria applicable to asbestos analytical laboratories;

5. Promulgate regulations governing the functions and duties of project monitors on asbestos projects, circumstances in which project monitors shall be required for asbestos projects, and training requirements for project monitors; and

6. Promulgate, in accordance with the Administrative Process Act, regulations necessary to establish procedures and requirements for the: (i) approval of lead-based paint activities training programs, (ii) licensure of individuals and firms to engage in lead inspection, evaluation, and abatement activities, and (iii) establishment of standards for performing lead-based paint activities consistent with the Residential Lead-based Paint Hazard Reduction Act and United States Environmental Protection

Agency regulations. If the United States Environmental Protection Agency (EPA) has adopted, prior to the promulgation of any related regulations by the Board, any final regulations relating to lead-based paint activities, then the related regulations of the Board shall not be more stringent than the EPA regulations in effect as of the date of such promulgation. In addition, if the EPA shall have outstanding any proposed regulations relating to lead-based paint activities (other than as amendments to existing EPA regulations), as of the date of promulgation of any related regulations by the board, then the related regulations of the Board shall not be more stringent than the proposed EPA regulations. In the event that the EPA shall adopt any final regulations subsequent to the promulgation by the Board of related regulations, then the Board shall, as soon as practicable, amend its existing regulations so as to be not more stringent than such EPA regulations.

§ 55-248.27

Rent escrow The tenant may assert that there exists upon the leased premises, a condition or conditions which constitute a material noncompliance by the landlord with the rental agreement or with provisions of law, or which if not promptly corrected, will constitute a fire hazard or serious threat to the life, health or safety of occupants thereof, including but not limited to, a lack of heat or hot or cold running water, except if the tenant is responsible for payment of the utility charge and where the lack of such heat or hot or cold running water is the direct result of the tenant's failure to pay the utility charge; or of light, electricity or adequate sewage disposal facilities; or an infestation of rodents, except if the property is a one-family dwelling; or of the existence of paint containing lead pigment on surfaces within the dwelling, provided that the landlord has notice of such paint. The tenant may file such an assertion in a general district court wherein the premises are located by a declaration setting forth such assertion and asking for one or more forms of relief as provided for in §55-248.29.

§ 55-519 Required Disclosures

A. With regard to transfers described in §55-517 of this chapter, the owner of the residential real property shall furnish to a purchaser one of the following:

1. A residential property disclaimer statement in a form provided by the Real Estate Board stating that the owner makes no

representations or warranties as to the condition of the real property or any improvements thereon, and that the purchaser will be receiving the real property "as is," that is, with all defects which may exist, if any, except as otherwise provided in the real estate purchase contract; or

2. A residential property disclosure statement disclosing those items contained in a form provided by the Real Estate Board to implement the provisions of this chapter and to list items which are required to be disclosed relative to the physical condition of the property. Such disclosure form may include defects of which the owner has actual knowledge regarding: (i) the water and sewer systems, including the source of household water, water treatment system, sprinkler system; (ii) insulation; (iii) structural systems, including roof, walls, floors, foundation and any basement; (iv) plumbing, electrical, heat and air conditioning systems; (v) wood-destroying insect infestation; (vi) land use matters; (vii) hazardous or regulated materials, including asbestos, lead-based paint, radon and underground storage tanks; and (viii)

other material defects known to the owner. The disclosure form shall contain a notice to prospective purchasers and owners that the prospective purchaser and the owner may wish to obtain professional advice or inspections of the property. The disclosure form shall also contain a notice to purchasers that the information contained in the disclosure is the representations of the owner and is not the representations of the broker or salesperson, if any. The owner shall not be required to undertake or provide any independent investigation or inspection of the property in order to make the disclosures required by this chapter.

B. The disclosure and disclaimer forms shall contain a notice to purchasers that regardless of whether the owner proceeds under subdivision 1 or 2, the owner makes no representations with respect to any matters which may pertain to parcels adjacent to the subject parcel. Further, such notice shall advise purchasers to exercise whatever due diligence a particular purchaser deems necessary with respect to adjacent parcels in accordance with terms and conditions as may be contained in the real estate purchase contract, but in any event, prior to settlement on a parcel of residential real property.

B. Any owner or any other person, firm or corporation violating any Code provisions relating to the removal or the covering of lead-based paint which poses a hazard to the health of pregnant women and children under the age of six years who occupy the premises shall, upon conviction, be guilty of a misdemeanor and shall be subject to a fine of not more than $2,500. If the court convicts pursuant to this subsection and sets a time by which such hazard must be abated, each day the hazard remains unabated after the time set for the abatement has expired shall constitute a separate violation of the Uniform Statewide Building Code. Upon a reasonable showing to the court by a landlord as defined in §55-248.4, that such landlord is financially unable to abate the lead-based paint hazard, the court shall order any rental agreement related to the affected premises terminated effective thirty days from the entry of the court order. For the purposes of the preceding sentence, termination of the rental agreement shall not be deemed noncompliance by the landlord pursuant to §55248.21.

§ 40.1-100 Certain employment prohibited or limited

A. No child under eighteen years of age shall be employed, permitted or suffered to work:

> 5. In any capacity in the manufacturing of paints, colors, white lead, or brick tile or kindred products, or in any place where goods of alcoholic content are manufactured, bottled, or sold for consumption on the premises except in places where the sale of alcoholic beverages is merely incidental to the main business actually conducted, or to deliver alcoholic goods;

Epilogue

My sincere thanks and appreciation to everyone who reads this book. It has been a work that required many hours of time that were not my own. My involvement in lead poisoning prevention is not a position that I sought or applied for. Instead, like many of us I was chosen for the mission.

Even today sometimes I feel so overwhelmed and question why I was chosen for this mission. At times I have to put my head in my hands and cry. I cry every time I read of the lead related deaths, of the children who are exposed today, children who will never live up to their fullest potential. I cry for the children of Flint, Michigan, Of the industries that to this day tries to downplay the seriousness of the matter. This industry that has megabucks to fight with to continuously tilt the scales of justice in their favor. I cry because we live in a capitalistic society that values money over quality of life and indeed life itself. I cry because, for the right price doctors and elected officials can be persuaded to go along with the industry's views and publish those views to a gullible public. If we hear or read something enough times coming from those in "respected" positions we will begin to believe it. I say to you, especially parents, don't be afraid to ask questions. Don't take anything at face value. Things are not always as they appear. On the days when I ask, "Lord why me?" How can I continue to fight when my arms are so weary? I am reminded of Moses standing up to the mighty Pharaoh and of the courageous Harriet Tubman who refused to turn back and my fears are calmed. My spirit is quickened and I am strengthened with the power of my Ancestors who overcame great odds. And the Lord answers, "Why not you?" I can hear the voices of my Ancestors saying "don't you know Allah is All Mighty and has never lost a battle." They say, "Tell the children to hold on Change is Coming."

Afterword by Cynthia Williams Mendy

Children are precious jewels and resources that should be handled delicately, lovingly and tenderly. All children deserve a healthy and fair start in life. They should also be protected from environmental harms, such as lead poisoning, which can impede their quality of life. Lead poisoning is the major environmental health threat to children in the United States, especially children ages 6 years and younger. The disease can affect all children; however, it disproportionately burdens African-American children and children of low income.

Contrary to the myth that lead poisoning is no longer a problem, children all across the United States continue to be threatened by this preventable disease. Lead poisoning threatens the life chance of many children and reduces the quality of life. The effects of the disease are devastating and irreversible. Even at low levels of exposure, lead poisoning is linked to a host of lead health problems, such as brain, hearing, and nerve damage, hyperactivity, developmental impairments, reduced cognition, hypertension, and sterility. High levels of lead in the body can cause seizures, comas, and death.

In A Child Is A Terrible Thing to Waste, Zakia Shabazz captures the reader's heart and mind with her vivid and touching account of her family's journey and battle to tackle lead poisoning and its consequences. Her story reminds one that lead poisoning has an array of ramifications that affect the lead poisoned child, the family, and society. The book is also a reminder of society's failure to protect all children from lead poisoning. In A Child Is A Terrible Thing to Waste, it is clear that Zakia's determination to protect all children from lead poisoning is unshakeable.

Protecting all children from lead poisoning is everyone's responsibility and requires public awareness, education, resources, commitment and action. Everyone must strive vigorously to annihilate barriers that prevent the eradication of lead poisoning. All children deserve healthy and safe environments. Eradication of lead poisoning is preservation of human life.

* * * * * * * *

Now Available for Bookings Nationwide

Queen Zakia Shabazz, Author
Founder/Executive Director
United Parents Against Lead
& Other Environmental Hazards (UPAL)
4809 Old Warwick Road
P.O. Box 24773
Richmond, Virginia 23224
Website: UPAL (upalnational.org)
Phone (804)308-1518
E-mail: unitedparentsagainstlead@gmail.com

Help us to bring about change for our children…

We Need Your Support Send your best gift to:

UPAL Foundation
For Lead Poisoned Children
P.O. Box 24773
Richmond, Virginia 23224

UPAL is a non-profit organization that depends on the free will gifts of support from friends like you.

Please help if you can.
Email Address and Phone (Optional)

Yes! I want to help the children who have been affected by lead. Here is my gfit:

___$25   ___$50   ___$100

___$500   ___$1,000   Other $___

Name:____________________________________

Address: _________________________________

City, State: Zip: __________________________

Share the story of **A Child is a Terrible Thing to Waste** with a friend. We believe that the more people are aware of the problems in society that are causing irreversible damage to so many of our children the sooner we can begin to address the problem. Our goals are to eradicate lead poisoning.

After you have read this book, please pass it along to a friend. Order copies to use as your organization's fundraiser. If you would like to purchase more copies just fill out the coupon below and return it to us.

You know that because you took the time to care a precious child will receive the benefits of a better life.

Name: _______________________________________

Address: _____________________________________

City, State: Zip: ______________________________

Please send me __________ copies of *A Child is a Terrible Thing to Waste:*

Enclosed is $17.00 per book, (Includes shipping & handling) Please allow six to eight weeks for your order to be processed and delivered.

Call UPAL at (804) 308-1518 for Wholesale/Fund Raiser Price List

*** COMING SOON * COMING SOON ***
*** COMING SOON * COMING SOON ***
*** COMING SOON ***

A GRAY PAPER

Breaking the Silence of Lead Poisoning Through
the Study of Lead and its Effect on People

Activity

By

Queen Zakia Rafiqa Shabazz

Back in 1999 I was asked to provide a quote for
the Introduction to a Community Resource Guide
for Lead Poisoning Prevention in California.

"Our children had no chance against the hidden
dangers of lead poison because no one had told us.
If someone did utter a few words about lead it was
so hushed and rushed that it was brushed off as
insignificant and certainly not something that was
placed at the top of our priorities list. Lead Awareness
Campaigns must state unequivocally that lead does
cause brain damage, learning disabilities, reduced
IQ in children. Parents want to protect our children

but we can do little against an invisible or unknown enemy"

In 2024 and beyond the enemy is no longer unknown, no longer invisible. A Gray Paper breaks the silence of lead poisoning and reveals what life is like for children who suffer with lead laden voices.

Triumphing Over Lead - Severing the Social Stigma will be released in 2025 and contains the first person narrative of Zaki Abdullah Shabazz. Zaki, as a lead poisoning survivor, shares his account of how lead impacted his life and how he ultimately triumphed over lead.

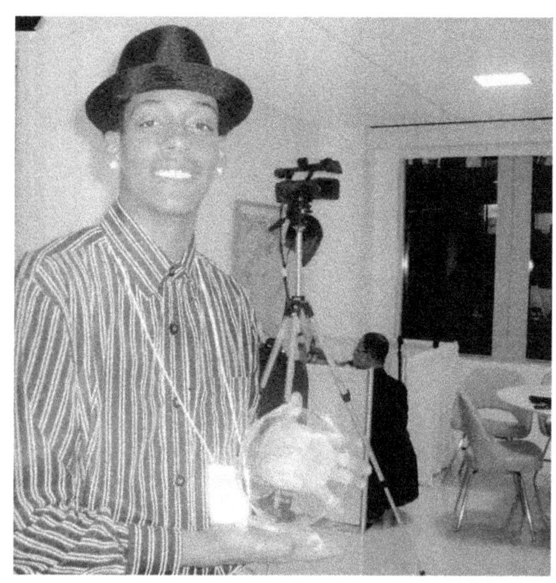

Zaki

A NEW BEGINNING